# Menopause Die
# for Women Over 50

Dr. Christie Barron

# Disclaimer

Please keep in mind that the content in this book is solely
for educational purposes. The information offered here is
said to be reliable and trustworthy. The author makes no
implication or intends to offer any warranty of accuracy for
particular individual cases.
Before beginning any diet or lifestyle habits, it is
recommended that you contact a knowledgeable
practitioner, such as your doctor. This book's material
should not be utilized in place of expert counsel or
professional guidance.
The author, publisher, and distributor expressly disclaim
all liability, loss, damage, or danger incurred by persons
who rely on the information in this book, whether directly
or indirectly.
All intellectual property rights are retained. This book's
information should not be replicated in any way,
mechanically, electronically, photocopying, or by any other
methods accessible

Copyright © Dr. Christie Barron

# Table of Contents

# Why You Should Give this Book a Chance

Are you experiencing the challenges that often accompany menopause, such as hormonal fluctuations, weight gain, and changes in metabolism? Do you find it challenging to maintain a balanced and nutritious diet during this transformative phase of life? If so, you're not alone. The menopausal journey can be both empowering and challenging, and your diet plays a pivotal role in navigating this transition successfully.

*But fear not—there is a solution tailored just for you.*

## Unlock the Power of Nutrition: Addressing Menopausal Challenges

Our book, "Menopause Diet Recipes for Women Over 50," is not just a cookbook; it's your guide to embracing menopause with vitality, addressing common concerns, and savoring delicious recipes crafted to meet your nutritional needs.

## Why Consider This Book?

### Hormone Harmony:
- **Challenge:** Hormonal imbalances during menopause can lead to mood swings and disrupted sleep.
- **Solution:** Explore recipes rich in nutrients known to support hormonal balance, promoting a smoother transition and enhanced well-being.

### Weight Management:
- **Challenge:** Menopause often brings changes in metabolism and weight gain.

- **Solution:** Our recipes focus on wholesome, nutrient-dense ingredients to support a healthy weight, offering a delicious way to manage and thrive.

**Bone Health:**
- **Challenge:** Decreased estrogen levels can impact bone density.
- **Solution:** Delve into recipes featuring calcium and vitamin D-rich foods, promoting bone health and resilience.

**Heart Health:**
- **Challenge:** Hormonal shifts can affect heart health.
- **Solution:** Explore heart-healthy recipes designed to support cardiovascular well-being, allowing you to enjoy meals that love your heart back.

**Mood Enhancement:**
- **Challenge:** Menopausal symptoms can affect mood and energy levels.
- **Solution:** Indulge in recipes featuring mood-boosting ingredients, helping you stay vibrant and energized.

**Gut Health:**
- **Challenge:** Digestive issues may arise during menopause.
- **Solution:** Our recipes incorporate fiber-rich foods to nurture your gut health, fostering overall digestive well-being.

**And much, much more...**

**What Sets This Book Apart?**
- **Variety and Flavor:** Enjoy 75 meticulously crafted recipes spanning breakfast, lunch, and dinner. Diverse and flavorful, these recipes make healthy eating a delight.
- **Nutritional Guidance:** Each recipe comes with detailed nutritional information, empowering you to make informed choices that align with your dietary needs.
- **Educational Insights:** Gain in-depth knowledge about the impact of nutrition on menopause. Understand the science behind each ingredient and its role in supporting your well-being.

**Embark on a Journey of Transformation:**

Your menopausal years should be a time of empowerment and celebration, and our book is your trusted companion on this transformative journey. "Menopause Diet Recipes for Women Over 50" isn't just a recipe collection—it's a holistic approach to well-being.

Are you ready to nourish your body, uplift your spirit, and savor every moment of this incredible chapter? If your answer is a resounding "yes," then this book is tailor-made for you. Embrace the power of nutrition and embark on a journey of vitality, balance, and joy.

Your best years are just a recipe away!

# RECIPES

# Quinoa Breakfast Bowl

**Intro:** This Quinoa Breakfast Bowl is a nutrient-packed way to start your day. Packed with protein, fiber, and a variety of textures, it's a delicious and satisfying breakfast option.

**Total Prep Time:** 20 minutes

## Ingredients:
- 1 cup cooked quinoa
- 1/2 cup Greek yogurt
- 1/2 cup mixed berries (strawberries, blueberries, raspberries)
- 1 tablespoon honey
- 2 tablespoons chopped nuts (almonds, walnuts)
- 1 teaspoon chia seeds

## Instructions:
1. In a bowl, layer the cooked quinoa.
2. Top with Greek yogurt and spread it evenly.
3. Add a layer of mixed berries on top.
4. Drizzle honey over the berries.
5. Sprinkle chopped nuts and chia seeds for added crunch.
6. Mix well before eating to combine all the flavors.

## Nutritional Information: (Per Serving)
- Calories: 350
- Protein: 15g
- Carbohydrates: 45g
- Fat: 12g
- Fiber: 8g

# Greek Yogurt Parfait with Berries

**Intro:** Indulge in a wholesome Greek Yogurt Parfait with Berries, a delightful combination of creamy yogurt, fresh berries, and crunchy granola. It's a quick and nutritious breakfast or snack.
**Total Prep Time:** 10 minutes

## Ingredients:
- 1 cup Greek yogurt
- 1/2 cup mixed berries (blueberries, strawberries)
- 1/4 cup granola
- 1 tablespoon honey
- 1 teaspoon flaxseeds

## Instructions:
1. In a glass or bowl, layer Greek yogurt at the bottom.
2. Add a layer of mixed berries.
3. Sprinkle granola evenly over the berries.
4. Drizzle honey on top for sweetness.
5. Garnish with flaxseeds for added nutrition.
6. Repeat layers and enjoy!

## Nutritional Information: (Per Serving)
- Calories: 280
- Protein: 18g
- Carbohydrates: 30g
- Fat: 10g
- Fiber: 5g

# Veggie Omelette with Spinach and Feta

**Intro:** Start your morning with a Veggie Omelette filled with nutrient-rich spinach and flavorful feta cheese. It's a protein-packed breakfast that will keep you energized throughout the day.

**Total Prep Time:** 15 minutes

## Ingredients:
- 2 eggs
- 1/2 cup fresh spinach, chopped
- 2 tablespoons feta cheese, crumbled
- 1/4 cup bell peppers, diced
- Salt and pepper to taste
- 1 tablespoon olive oil

## Instructions:
1. In a bowl, beat the eggs and season with salt and pepper.
2. Heat olive oil in a pan over medium heat.
3. Add bell peppers and sauté until slightly softened.
4. Add chopped spinach to the pan and cook until wilted.
5. Pour the beaten eggs over the veggies.
6. Sprinkle crumbled feta over the eggs.
7. Cook until the edges set, then fold the omelette in half.
8. Cook until eggs are fully set. Serve hot.

## Nutritional Information: (Per Serving)
- Calories: 280
- Protein: 15g
- Carbohydrates: 4g
- Fat: 22g
- Fiber: 2g

# Chia Seed Pudding with Almonds and Berries

**Intro:** This Chia Seed Pudding with Almonds and Berries is a delightful make-ahead breakfast option. Packed with omega-3 fatty acids, fiber, and antioxidants, it's a nutritious way to kickstart your day.

**Total Prep Time:** 5 minutes (plus overnight chilling)

## Ingredients:
- 3 tablespoons chia seeds
- 1 cup almond milk
- 1/2 teaspoon vanilla extract
- 1 tablespoon honey
- 2 tablespoons sliced almonds
- 1/2 cup mixed berries

## Instructions:
1. In a jar, combine chia seeds, almond milk, and vanilla extract.
2. Stir well, then refrigerate overnight or for at least 4 hours.
3. Before serving, drizzle honey over the chia pudding.
4. Top with sliced almonds and mixed berries.
5. Stir gently and enjoy this nutritious and delicious pudding.

## Nutritional Information: (Per Serving)
- Calories: 220
- Protein: 7g
- Carbohydrates: 25g
- Fat: 12g
- Fiber: 10g

# Avocado Toast with Smoked Salmon

**Intro:** Elevate your breakfast with this Avocado Toast with Smoked Salmon. Creamy avocado, smoked salmon, and a hint of lemon create a delicious and satisfying morning meal.

**Total Prep Time:** 10 minutes

## Ingredients:
- 1 slice whole grain bread, toasted
- 1/2 ripe avocado, mashed
- 2 ounces smoked salmon
- 1 teaspoon capers
- Lemon wedge for squeezing
- Fresh dill for garnish

## Instructions:
1. Toast the whole grain bread to your liking.
2. Spread mashed avocado evenly over the toast.
3. Drape smoked salmon over the avocado.
4. Sprinkle capers on top.
5. Squeeze fresh lemon juice over the salmon.
6. Garnish with fresh dill.
7. Serve immediately and savor the flavors.

## Nutritional Information: (Per Serving)
- Calories: 280
- Protein: 20g
- Carbohydrates: 20g
- Fat: 15g
- Fiber: 8g

# Blueberry Banana Smoothie

**Intro:** This Blueberry Banana Smoothie is a refreshing and nutritious way to start your day. Packed with antioxidants, vitamins, and minerals, it's a delicious choice for a quick breakfast.

**Total Prep Time:** 5 minutes

## Ingredients:
- 1 cup blueberries
- 1 banana, peeled
- 1/2 cup Greek yogurt
- 1/2 cup almond milk
- 1 tablespoon honey
- Ice cubes (optional)

## Instructions:
1. In a blender, combine blueberries, banana, Greek yogurt, and almond milk.
2. Blend until smooth and creamy.
3. Add honey for sweetness and blend again.
4. If desired, add ice cubes and blend until well combined.
5. Pour into a glass and enjoy this vibrant and nutritious smoothie.

## Nutritional Information: (Per Serving)
- Calories: 200
- Protein: 10g
- Carbohydrates: 40g
- Fat: 3g
- Fiber: 6g

# Whole Grain Pancakes with Maple Syrup

**Intro:** These Whole Grain Pancakes with Maple Syrup are a wholesome twist on a classic breakfast. Made with whole grains and topped with pure maple syrup, they are a delicious and satisfying morning treat.
**Total Prep Time:** 20 minutes

## Ingredients:
- 1 cup whole wheat flour
- 1/2 cup oats
- 2 teaspoons baking powder
- 1/2 teaspoon cinnamon
- 1 cup milk
- 1 egg
- 2 tablespoons maple syrup
- 1 teaspoon vanilla extract
- Cooking spray or butter for the pan

## Instructions:
1. In a bowl, whisk together whole wheat flour, oats, baking powder, and cinnamon.
2. In a separate bowl, whisk together milk, egg, maple syrup, and vanilla extract.
3. Pour the wet ingredients into the dry ingredients and stir until just combined.
4. Heat a griddle or pan over medium heat and coat with cooking spray or butter.
5. Pour 1/4 cup of batter for each pancake onto the griddle.
6. Cook until bubbles form on the surface, then flip and cook until golden brown.
7. Serve hot with a drizzle of maple syrup.

**Nutritional Information:** (Per Serving, 2 pancakes)
- Calories: 300
- Protein: 10g
- Carbohydrates: 55g
- Fat: 5g
- Fiber: 8g

# Sweet Potato and Kale Hash

**Intro:** This Sweet Potato and Kale Hash is a nutrient-dense and flavorful breakfast option. Packed with vitamins and minerals, it's a delicious way to incorporate veggies into your morning routine.
**Total Prep Time:** 25 minutes

## Ingredients:
- 1 sweet potato, diced
- 1 cup kale, chopped
- 1/2 onion, diced
- 2 cloves garlic, minced
- 2 tablespoons olive oil
- Salt and pepper to taste
- 1/4 teaspoon paprika
- 2 eggs (optional, for serving)

## Instructions:
1. Heat olive oil in a skillet over medium heat.
2. Add diced sweet potato and cook until slightly browned and softened.
3. Add diced onion and minced garlic, sauté until fragrant.
4. Stir in chopped kale and cook until wilted.
5. Season with salt, pepper, and paprika.

6. If desired, fry or poach eggs and place them on top of the hash.
7. Serve hot, and enjoy a nutrient-packed breakfast.

**Nutritional Information:** (Per Serving)
- Calories: 250
- Protein: 8g
- Carbohydrates: 30g
- Fat: 12g
- Fiber: 5g

# Almond Butter and Banana Wrap

**Intro:** This Almond Butter and Banana Wrap is a quick and satisfying breakfast option, combining the natural sweetness of bananas with the richness of almond butter in a convenient wrap.

**Total Prep Time:** 10 minutes

**Ingredients:**
- 1 whole wheat wrap
- 2 tablespoons almond butter
- 1 banana, sliced
- 1 teaspoon honey
- 1 tablespoon chopped almonds

**Instructions:**
1. Spread almond butter evenly over the whole wheat wrap.
2. Place banana slices in the center of the wrap.
3. Drizzle honey over the bananas.
4. Sprinkle chopped almonds on top.
5. Fold the sides of the wrap and roll it tightly.

6.  Slice in half if desired and enjoy this delicious and portable breakfast.

**Nutritional Information:** (Per Serving)
- Calories: 380
- Protein: 8g
- Carbohydrates: 45g
- Fat: 20g
- Fiber: 7g

# Spinach and Mushroom Breakfast Quesadilla

**Intro:** Spice up your morning with this Spinach and Mushroom Breakfast Quesadilla. Filled with sautéed veggies, cheese, and eggs, it's a tasty and satisfying way to start the day.

**Total Prep Time:** 15 minutes

**Ingredients:**
- 2 whole wheat tortillas
- 1 cup fresh spinach
- 1/2 cup mushrooms, sliced
- 2 eggs, beaten
- 1/2 cup shredded mozzarella cheese
- Salt and pepper to taste
- Cooking spray or olive oil for the pan
- Salsa and Greek yogurt for serving (optional)

**Instructions:**
1.  In a pan, sauté sliced mushrooms until golden brown.
2.  Add fresh spinach and cook until wilted.
3.  Remove veggies from the pan and set aside.

4. In the same pan, pour beaten eggs and scramble until cooked.
5. Place a tortilla in the pan, add a layer of scrambled eggs, sautéed veggies, and mozzarella cheese.
6. Top with the second tortilla and press down gently.
7. Cook until the tortilla is golden brown, then flip and cook the other side.
8. Remove from the pan, slice, and serve with salsa and Greek yogurt if desired.

**Nutritional Information:** (Per Serving)
- Calories: 400
- Protein: 20g
- Carbohydrates: 30g
- Fat: 22g
- Fiber: 6g

## Coconut Yogurt with Granola and Mango

**Intro:** Start your day with a tropical twist! This Coconut Yogurt with Granola and Mango is a refreshing and nutritious breakfast option that combines the creamy goodness of coconut yogurt with the crunch of granola and the sweetness of ripe mango.

**Total Prep Time:** 10 minutes

**Ingredients:**
- 1 cup coconut yogurt
- 1/2 cup granola
- 1/2 mango, diced
- 1 tablespoon shredded coconut (optional)
- Drizzle of honey (optional)

## Instructions:
1. In a bowl, spoon coconut yogurt as the base.
2. Sprinkle granola evenly over the yogurt.
3. Top with diced mango for a burst of sweetness.
4. Optional: Sprinkle shredded coconut on top.
5. Drizzle honey for extra sweetness.
6. Mix gently and enjoy this tropical delight.

## Nutritional Information: (Per Serving)
- Calories: 300
- Protein: 8g
- Carbohydrates: 45g
- Fat: 10g
- Fiber: 6g

# Egg and Vegetable Muffins

**Intro:** These Egg and Vegetable Muffins are a convenient and protein-packed breakfast option. Packed with colorful veggies and protein-rich eggs, they are perfect for meal prep and can be enjoyed on the go.
**Total Prep Time:** 25 minutes

## Ingredients:
- 6 eggs
- 1/2 cup bell peppers, diced
- 1/2 cup cherry tomatoes, halved
- 1/4 cup red onion, finely chopped
- 1/4 cup spinach, chopped
- Salt and pepper to taste
- 1/2 cup shredded cheese (optional)

**Instructions:**

1. Preheat the oven to 350°F (175°C) and grease a muffin tin.
2. In a bowl, whisk together eggs, salt, and pepper.
3. Stir in diced bell peppers, cherry tomatoes, red onion, and chopped spinach.
4. Pour the egg mixture evenly into the muffin cups.
5. Optional: Sprinkle shredded cheese on top.
6. Bake for 15-20 minutes or until the eggs are set.
7. Allow to cool slightly before removing from the muffin tin.
8. Serve warm and enjoy these veggie-packed muffins.

**Nutritional Information:** (Per Serving, 2 muffins)

- Calories: 180
- Protein: 14g
- Carbohydrates: 6g
- Fat: 12g
- Fiber: 2g

# Overnight Oats with Mixed Nuts and Dried Fruit

**Intro:** Simplify your mornings with these Overnight Oats with Mixed Nuts and Dried Fruit. Prep the night before for a quick and delicious breakfast that's loaded with fiber, protein, and a variety of textures.

**Total Prep Time:** 5 minutes (plus overnight chilling)

**Ingredients:**

- 1/2 cup rolled oats
- 1/2 cup milk (dairy or plant-based)
- 1 tablespoon chia seeds
- 2 tablespoons mixed nuts (almonds, walnuts)

- 2 tablespoons dried fruit (raisins, cranberries)
- 1 tablespoon honey or maple syrup

**Instructions:**
1. In a jar or bowl, combine rolled oats, milk, and chia seeds.
2. Stir well and refrigerate overnight or for at least 4 hours.
3. Before serving, top with mixed nuts and dried fruit.
4. Drizzle honey or maple syrup for sweetness.
5. Stir gently and enjoy these hearty and nutritious overnight oats.

**Nutritional Information:** (Per Serving)
- Calories: 320
- Protein: 10g
- Carbohydrates: 40g
- Fat: 15g
- Fiber: 8g

## Smashed Avocado on Whole Grain Toast

**Intro:** Simple yet satisfying, Smashed Avocado on Whole Grain Toast is a classic breakfast choice. Creamy avocado meets crunchy whole grain toast for a delightful combination that's rich in healthy fats and fiber.
**Total Prep Time:** 5 minutes

**Ingredients:**
- 1 ripe avocado
- 2 slices whole grain bread, toasted
- Salt and pepper to taste
- Red pepper flakes (optional)
- Lemon wedge for squeezing

## Instructions:
1. Toast the whole grain bread to your liking.
2. Cut the ripe avocado in half and remove the pit.
3. Scoop the avocado into a bowl and mash it with a fork.
4. Spread the smashed avocado evenly over the toasted bread.
5. Season with salt, pepper, and red pepper flakes if desired.
6. Squeeze fresh lemon juice over the top.
7. Serve immediately and savor this quick and nourishing breakfast.

## Nutritional Information: (Per Serving)
- Calories: 280
- Protein: 6g
- Carbohydrates: 25g
- Fat: 18g
- Fiber: 8g

# Salmon and Cream Cheese Bagel

**Intro:** Elevate your breakfast with this Salmon and Cream Cheese Bagel. Smoked salmon, creamy cheese, and fresh herbs create a flavorful combination that's perfect for a leisurely morning or a special occasion.
**Total Prep Time:** 10 minutes

## Ingredients:
- 1 whole grain or everything bagel, sliced and toasted
- 2 ounces smoked salmon
- 2 tablespoons cream cheese
- Red onion slices

- Capers
- Fresh dill for garnish
- Lemon wedge for serving

## Instructions:

1. Toast the bagel slices to your liking.
2. Spread cream cheese evenly over each bagel half.
3. Place smoked salmon on top of the cream cheese.
4. Add red onion slices and capers for extra flavor.
5. Garnish with fresh dill.
6. Serve with a wedge of lemon on the side.
7. Enjoy this delightful and elegant breakfast.

## Nutritional Information: (Per Serving)

- Calories: 350
- Protein: 18g
- Carbohydrates: 30g
- Fat: 18g
- Fiber: 4g

# Berry Protein Smoothie Bowl

**Intro:** Power up your morning with a Berry Protein Smoothie Bowl. Packed with antioxidants, protein, and natural sweetness, this vibrant bowl is a delicious way to fuel your day.

**Total Prep Time:** 10 minutes

## Ingredients:

- 1 cup mixed berries (strawberries, blueberries, raspberries)
- 1/2 banana, frozen
- 1/2 cup Greek yogurt
- 1 scoop vanilla protein powder

- 1/4 cup almond milk
- Toppings: granola, sliced almonds, chia seeds, fresh berries

## Instructions:

1. In a blender, combine mixed berries, frozen banana, Greek yogurt, protein powder, and almond milk.
2. Blend until smooth and creamy.
3. Pour the smoothie into a bowl.
4. Top with granola, sliced almonds, chia seeds, and fresh berries.
5. Customize with your favorite toppings.
6. Enjoy this nutrient-packed and satisfying smoothie bowl.

## Nutritional Information: (Per Serving)

- Calories: 400
- Protein: 25g
- Carbohydrates: 50g
- Fat: 12g
- Fiber: 10g

# Breakfast Burrito with Black Beans and Salsa

**Intro:** Spice up your morning with this Breakfast Burrito filled with black beans, eggs, and flavorful salsa. It's a protein-packed, satisfying, and convenient option for a hearty breakfast.

**Total Prep Time:** 20 minutes

## Ingredients:

- 1 large whole wheat tortilla

- 2 eggs, scrambled
- 1/2 cup black beans, cooked and drained
- 1/4 cup shredded cheddar cheese
- 2 tablespoons salsa
- Avocado slices for garnish (optional)
- Fresh cilantro for garnish (optional)

## Instructions:
1. In a pan, scramble the eggs until cooked.
2. Warm the tortilla in a dry pan or microwave.
3. Place the scrambled eggs in the center of the tortilla.
4. Add black beans, shredded cheddar cheese, and salsa.
5. Optional: Garnish with avocado slices and fresh cilantro.
6. Fold the sides of the tortilla and roll it into a burrito.
7. Serve hot and enjoy this flavorful breakfast.

## Nutritional Information: (Per Serving)
- Calories: 420
- Protein: 22g
- Carbohydrates: 40g
- Fat: 18g
- Fiber: 10g

# Pumpkin Spice Quinoa Porridge

**Intro:** Embrace the fall flavors with this Pumpkin Spice Quinoa Porridge. Packed with protein, fiber, and the warm spices of pumpkin, cinnamon, and nutmeg, it's a comforting and nutritious breakfast option.

**Total Prep Time:** 20 minutes

## Ingredients:

- 1/2 cup quinoa, rinsed
- 1 cup almond milk
- 1/4 cup canned pumpkin puree
- 1 tablespoon maple syrup
- 1/2 teaspoon pumpkin pie spice (or a mix of cinnamon, nutmeg, and cloves)
- 1/4 cup chopped pecans
- Dried cranberries for garnish

## Instructions:

1. In a saucepan, combine quinoa and almond milk.
2. Bring to a boil, then reduce heat and simmer until quinoa is cooked.
3. Stir in pumpkin puree, maple syrup, and pumpkin pie spice.
4. Cook for an additional 5 minutes, stirring occasionally.
5. Remove from heat and let it sit for a few minutes to thicken.
6. Serve the quinoa porridge in bowls.
7. Top with chopped pecans and dried cranberries.
8. Enjoy this cozy and nutritious pumpkin spice breakfast.

## Nutritional Information: (Per Serving)

- Calories: 350
- Protein: 10g
- Carbohydrates: 50g
- Fat: 12g
- Fiber: 8g

# Mediterranean Frittata with Olives and Tomatoes

**Intro:** Transport yourself to the Mediterranean with this flavorful Frittata. Loaded with olives, tomatoes, and feta cheese, it's a protein-rich and satisfying breakfast that's bursting with Mediterranean flavors.

**Total Prep Time:** 25 minutes

## Ingredients:
- 6 eggs
- 1/2 cup cherry tomatoes, halved
- 1/4 cup Kalamata olives, pitted and sliced
- 1/4 cup feta cheese, crumbled
- 1/4 cup fresh basil, chopped
- Salt and pepper to taste
- 1 tablespoon olive oil

## Instructions:
1. Preheat the oven to 375°F (190°C).
2. In a bowl, beat the eggs and season with salt and pepper.
3. Heat olive oil in an oven-safe skillet over medium heat.
4. Add cherry tomatoes and cook until softened.
5. Stir in olives and feta cheese.
6. Pour the beaten eggs over the veggies and let it set for a minute.
7. Sprinkle fresh basil on top.
8. Transfer the skillet to the preheated oven and bake until the frittata is set and slightly golden.
9. Remove from the oven, slice, and serve.

**Nutritional Information:** (Per Serving)
- Calories: 280
- Protein: 18g
- Carbohydrates: 6g
- Fat: 20g
- Fiber: 2g

# Apple Cinnamon Quinoa Bowl

**Intro:** Kickstart your morning with this Apple Cinnamon Quinoa Bowl. Packed with the goodness of quinoa, fresh apples, and warm cinnamon, it's a hearty and flavorful breakfast that will keep you satisfied.
**Total Prep Time:** 20 minutes

**Ingredients:**
- 1/2 cup quinoa, rinsed
- 1 cup water
- 1 apple, diced
- 1 tablespoon almond butter
- 1 teaspoon honey
- 1/2 teaspoon cinnamon
- Chopped nuts for garnish (walnuts or almonds)

**Instructions:**
1. In a saucepan, combine quinoa and water. Bring to a boil, then reduce heat and simmer until quinoa is cooked.
2. In a bowl, mix cooked quinoa, diced apple, almond butter, honey, and cinnamon.
3. Stir until well combined.
4. Optionally, top with chopped nuts for added crunch.

5. Serve warm and enjoy this wholesome and delicious quinoa bowl.

**Nutritional Information:** (Per Serving)
- Calories: 320
- Protein: 8g
- Carbohydrates: 55g
- Fat: 8g
- Fiber: 7g

# Veggie Breakfast Skewers

**Intro:** These Veggie Breakfast Skewers are a colorful and flavorful way to start your day. Packed with a variety of fresh vegetables, these skewers are not only delicious but also rich in vitamins and antioxidants.

**Total Prep Time:** 15 minutes

**Ingredients:**
- Cherry tomatoes
- Bell peppers (assorted colors), cut into chunks
- Zucchini, sliced
- Mushrooms, whole or halved
- Red onion, cut into chunks
- Olive oil
- Salt and pepper to taste
- Fresh herbs for garnish (optional)

**Instructions:**
1. Preheat the grill or grill pan.
2. Thread the vegetables onto skewers, alternating colors for a vibrant presentation.
3. Brush the skewers with olive oil and season with salt and pepper.

4. Grill for about 8-10 minutes, turning occasionally, until the veggies are tender and slightly charred.
5. Garnish with fresh herbs if desired.
6. Serve hot and enjoy these delightful Veggie Breakfast Skewers.

**Nutritional Information:** (Per Serving)
- Calories: 80
- Protein: 2g
- Carbohydrates: 10g
- Fat: 4g
- Fiber: 3g

# Green Tea Smoothie with Spinach and Pineapple

**Intro:** Boost your morning with this Green Tea Smoothie featuring the goodness of spinach and tropical sweetness from pineapple. Packed with antioxidants and nutrients, it's a refreshing and nutritious way to kickstart your day.
**Total Prep Time:** 10 minutes

**Ingredients:**
- 1 cup green tea, brewed and cooled
- 1 cup fresh spinach leaves
- 1/2 cup pineapple chunks
- 1 banana, frozen
- 1/2 cup Greek yogurt
- Honey or maple syrup to taste
- Ice cubes (optional)

**Instructions:**
1. Brew green tea and let it cool.

2. In a blender, combine green tea, fresh spinach, pineapple chunks, frozen banana, and Greek yogurt.
3. Blend until smooth.
4. Sweeten with honey or maple syrup to taste.
5. Add ice cubes if you prefer a colder smoothie.
6. Pour into a glass and enjoy this vibrant and energizing Green Tea Smoothie.

**Nutritional Information:** (Per Serving)
- Calories: 150
- Protein: 5g
- Carbohydrates: 30g
- Fat: 2g
- Fiber: 4g

# Cottage Cheese and Pineapple Bowl

**Intro:** This Cottage Cheese and Pineapple Bowl is a simple and satisfying breakfast that combines the creaminess of cottage cheese with the sweetness of fresh pineapple. It's a quick and nutritious way to start your day.
**Total Prep Time:** 5 minutes

**Ingredients:**
- 1 cup cottage cheese
- 1 cup fresh pineapple chunks
- Chopped mint or basil for garnish (optional)
- Drizzle of honey (optional)

**Instructions:**
1. Spoon cottage cheese into a bowl.
2. Top with fresh pineapple chunks.
3. Garnish with chopped mint or basil if desired.

4. Optional: Drizzle honey over the top for extra sweetness.
5. Mix gently and enjoy this easy and delicious Cottage Cheese and Pineapple Bowl.

**Nutritional Information:** (Per Serving)
- Calories: 220
- Protein: 20g
- Carbohydrates: 25g
- Fat: 4g
- Fiber: 2g

## Peanut Butter and Banana Breakfast Wrap

**Intro:** Wrap up your morning with this Peanut Butter and Banana Breakfast Wrap. A perfect balance of protein and natural sweetness, this wrap is a quick and satisfying option for a busy day.
**Total Prep Time:** 10 minutes

**Ingredients:**
- 1 whole wheat wrap
- 2 tablespoons peanut butter
- 1 banana, sliced
- 1 tablespoon honey
- 1 tablespoon chopped nuts (almonds, walnuts)

**Instructions:**
1. Spread peanut butter evenly over the whole wheat wrap.
2. Place banana slices in the center of the wrap.
3. Drizzle honey over the bananas.
4. Sprinkle chopped nuts on top.
5. Fold the sides of the wrap and roll it tightly.

6. Slice in half if desired and enjoy this delicious and portable Peanut Butter and Banana Breakfast Wrap.

**Nutritional Information:** (Per Serving)
- Calories: 380
- Protein: 10g
- Carbohydrates: 45g
- Fat: 20g
- Fiber: 7g

# Shakshuka with Spinach and Feta

**Intro:** Dive into a Mediterranean breakfast with this Shakshuka featuring spinach and feta. The rich and savory tomato sauce combined with poached eggs creates a hearty and flavorful dish that's perfect for brunch or any time of the day.

**Total Prep Time:** 30 minutes

**Ingredients:**
- 1 tablespoon olive oil
- 1 onion, diced
- 2 cloves garlic, minced
- 1 bell pepper, diced
- 1 teaspoon ground cumin
- 1 teaspoon smoked paprika
- 1/2 teaspoon cayenne pepper (optional, for heat)
- 1 can (14 oz) crushed tomatoes
- 2 cups fresh spinach leaves
- Salt and pepper to taste
- 4-6 eggs
- Feta cheese, crumbled, for garnish
- Fresh parsley, chopped, for garnish

- Crusty bread for serving

**Instructions:**
1. Heat olive oil in a large skillet over medium heat.
2. Sauté diced onion until softened.
3. Add minced garlic and diced bell pepper, cook until fragrant.
4. Stir in ground cumin, smoked paprika, and cayenne pepper (if using).
5. Pour in crushed tomatoes and simmer for 10-15 minutes.
6. Add fresh spinach, season with salt and pepper, and cook until wilted.
7. Create small wells in the sauce and crack eggs into them.
8. Cover the skillet and poach the eggs for 5-7 minutes or until the whites are set.
9. Garnish with crumbled feta and chopped parsley.
10. Serve hot with crusty bread for dipping.

**Nutritional Information:** (Per Serving, without bread)
- Calories: 180
- Protein: 10g
- Carbohydrates: 15g
- Fat: 10g
- Fiber: 5g

# Grilled Chicken Salad with Avocado and Quinoa

**Intro:** This Grilled Chicken Salad with Avocado and Quinoa is a satisfying and nutritious meal that combines the flavors of grilled chicken, creamy avocado, and wholesome quinoa. It's a perfect choice for a light and flavorful lunch or dinner.

**Total Prep Time:** 30 minutes

## Ingredients:

- 2 boneless, skinless chicken breasts
- 1 cup quinoa, cooked
- 2 cups mixed salad greens
- 1 avocado, sliced
- Cherry tomatoes, halved
- Cucumber, sliced
- Red onion, thinly sliced
- Olive oil and balsamic vinegar for dressing
- Salt and pepper to taste

## Instructions:

1. Season chicken breasts with salt and pepper, then grill until fully cooked. Slice into strips.
2. In a large bowl, combine cooked quinoa, salad greens, avocado slices, cherry tomatoes, cucumber, and red onion.
3. Add grilled chicken strips to the salad.
4. Drizzle with olive oil and balsamic vinegar, tossing to coat evenly.
5. Serve immediately and enjoy this wholesome Grilled Chicken Salad.

## Nutritional Information: (Per Serving)

- Calories: 400
- Protein: 25g
- Carbohydrates: 30g
- Fat: 20g
- Fiber: 8g

# Quinoa and Black Bean Stuffed Peppers

**Intro:** These Quinoa and Black Bean Stuffed Peppers are a flavorful and protein-packed vegetarian dish. Filled with a hearty mixture of quinoa, black beans, vegetables, and spices, they make for a delicious and wholesome meal.
**Total Prep Time:** 45 minutes

## Ingredients:
- 4 large bell peppers, halved and seeds removed
- 1 cup quinoa, cooked
- 1 can (15 oz) black beans, drained and rinsed
- 1 cup corn kernels (fresh or frozen)
- 1 cup diced tomatoes
- 1 cup shredded cheddar cheese
- 1 teaspoon cumin
- 1 teaspoon chili powder
- Salt and pepper to taste
- Fresh cilantro for garnish

## Instructions:
1. Preheat the oven to 375°F (190°C).
2. In a bowl, combine cooked quinoa, black beans, corn, diced tomatoes, shredded cheddar, cumin, chili powder, salt, and pepper.
3. Stuff each bell pepper half with the quinoa mixture.
4. Place the stuffed peppers in a baking dish.
5. Bake for 25-30 minutes or until the peppers are tender.
6. Garnish with fresh cilantro before serving.

**Nutritional Information:** (Per Serving, 1 stuffed pepper)
- Calories: 300

- Protein: 15g
- Carbohydrates: 40g
- Fat: 10g
- Fiber: 8g

# Greek Salad with Salmon

**Intro:** Elevate your salad game with this Greek Salad featuring grilled salmon. Bursting with Mediterranean flavors, this salad is a delightful combination of crisp vegetables, olives, feta cheese, and succulent salmon.
**Total Prep Time:** 20 minutes

## Ingredients:
- 1 lb salmon fillets
- 6 cups mixed salad greens
- Cherry tomatoes, halved
- Cucumber, sliced
- Red onion, thinly sliced
- Kalamata olives
- Feta cheese, crumbled
- Olive oil and red wine vinegar for dressing
- Oregano and black pepper to taste
- Lemon wedges for serving

## Instructions:
1. Season salmon fillets with olive oil, oregano, and black pepper.
2. Grill salmon until fully cooked, then flake into bite-sized pieces.
3. In a large bowl, combine salad greens, cherry tomatoes, cucumber, red onion, olives, and feta cheese.
4. Add grilled salmon to the salad.

5. Drizzle with olive oil and red wine vinegar, tossing gently.
6. Serve with lemon wedges for an extra burst of flavor.

**Nutritional Information:** (Per Serving)
- Calories: 400
- Protein: 30g
- Carbohydrates: 15g
- Fat: 25g
- Fiber: 5g

# Lentil and Vegetable Soup

**Intro:** Warm up with a bowl of hearty Lentil and Vegetable Soup. Packed with nutritious lentils, a medley of vegetables, and savory herbs, this soup is a comforting and wholesome option for a satisfying meal.
**Total Prep Time:** 45 minutes

**Ingredients:**
- 1 cup dried green or brown lentils, rinsed
- 1 onion, diced
- 2 carrots, diced
- 2 celery stalks, diced
- 3 cloves garlic, minced
- 1 can (14 oz) diced tomatoes
- 6 cups vegetable broth
- 1 teaspoon cumin
- 1 teaspoon coriander
- 1/2 teaspoon smoked paprika
- Salt and pepper to taste
- Fresh parsley for garnish

**Instructions:**
1. In a large pot, sauté diced onion, carrots, and celery until softened.
2. Add minced garlic and cook for an additional minute.
3. Stir in lentils, diced tomatoes, vegetable broth, cumin, coriander, smoked paprika, salt, and pepper.
4. Bring the soup to a boil, then reduce heat and simmer for 30-35 minutes or until lentils are tender.
5. Adjust seasoning as needed.
6. Garnish with fresh parsley before serving.

**Nutritional Information:** (Per Serving)
- Calories: 250
- Protein: 15g
- Carbohydrates: 40g
- Fat: 2g
- Fiber: 15g

# Turkey and Avocado Wrap

**Intro:** Enjoy a quick and satisfying lunch with this Turkey and Avocado Wrap. Packed with lean turkey, creamy avocado, crisp vegetables, and a zesty dressing, it's a delicious and balanced option for busy days.
**Total Prep Time:** 15 minutes

**Ingredients:**
- 1 large whole wheat wrap
- 4 oz sliced turkey breast
- 1/2 avocado, sliced
- 1/2 cup cherry tomatoes, halved

- 1/4 cup cucumber, thinly sliced
- 1/4 cup red onion, thinly sliced
- Lettuce leaves
- Greek yogurt or light mayo for dressing
- Salt and pepper to taste

**Instructions:**
1. Lay the whole wheat wrap on a flat surface.
2. Layer sliced turkey, avocado, cherry tomatoes, cucumber, red onion, and lettuce leaves.
3. Drizzle with Greek yogurt or light mayo.
4. Season with salt and pepper to taste.
5. Fold the sides of the wrap and roll it tightly.
6. Slice in half if desired and enjoy this Turkey and Avocado Wrap.

**Nutritional Information:** (Per Serving)
- Calories: 350
- Protein: 25g
- Carbohydrates: 30g
- Fat: 15g
- Fiber: 8g

## Spinach and Strawberry Salad with Balsamic Vinaigrette

**Intro:** Indulge in the sweetness of strawberries and the freshness of spinach with this delightful Spinach and Strawberry Salad. Tossed in a tangy balsamic vinaigrette, it's a vibrant and nutritious salad that's perfect for spring or summer.

**Total Prep Time:** 15 minutes

**Ingredients:**
- 4 cups fresh baby spinach
- 1 cup strawberries, sliced
- 1/4 cup feta cheese, crumbled
- 1/4 cup sliced almonds, toasted
- Balsamic vinaigrette dressing

**Instructions:**
1. In a large bowl, combine fresh baby spinach, sliced strawberries, crumbled feta, and toasted sliced almonds.
2. Drizzle with balsamic vinaigrette dressing and toss gently to coat.
3. Serve immediately, savoring the sweetness and crunch of this Spinach and Strawberry Salad.

**Nutritional Information:** (Per Serving)
- Calories: 200
- Protein: 7g
- Carbohydrates: 15g
- Fat: 14g
- Fiber: 5g

# Chickpea and Roasted Vegetable Buddha Bowl

**Intro:** Dive into a bowl of goodness with this Chickpea and Roasted Vegetable Buddha Bowl. Packed with protein, fiber, and a variety of textures, this bowl is a wholesome and satisfying meal that's easy to customize.

**Total Prep Time:** 40 minutes

**Ingredients:**
- 1 can (15 oz) chickpeas, drained and rinsed
- Assorted vegetables (e.g., sweet potatoes, broccoli, bell peppers), chopped
- Olive oil
- 1 teaspoon cumin
- 1 teaspoon paprika
- Salt and pepper to taste
- Quinoa or brown rice, cooked
- Avocado slices
- Hummus for dressing
- Fresh herbs for garnish (optional)

**Instructions:**
1. Preheat the oven to 400°F (200°C).
2. Toss chickpeas and chopped vegetables with olive oil, cumin, paprika, salt, and pepper.
3. Spread the mixture on a baking sheet and roast for 25-30 minutes or until vegetables are tender.
4. Assemble bowls with cooked quinoa or brown rice, roasted chickpeas and vegetables, avocado slices, and a dollop of hummus.
5. Garnish with fresh herbs if desired.
6. Enjoy this nourishing Chickpea and Roasted Vegetable Buddha Bowl.

**Nutritional Information:** (Per Serving)
- Calories: 400
- Protein: 15g
- Carbohydrates: 60g
- Fat: 12g
- Fiber: 12g

# Shrimp and Quinoa Salad

**Intro:** Refresh your palate with this Shrimp and Quinoa Salad. Packed with protein-rich shrimp, nutritious quinoa, and a medley of vegetables, it's a light and flavorful salad that's perfect for a satisfying lunch or dinner.

**Total Prep Time:** 25 minutes

## Ingredients:
- 1 cup quinoa, cooked
- 1 lb shrimp, peeled and deveined
- Cherry tomatoes, halved
- Cucumber, diced
- Red bell pepper, diced
- Avocado, sliced
- Fresh cilantro for garnish
- Lime wedges for serving
- Olive oil and lime juice for dressing
- Salt and pepper to taste

## Instructions:
1. Season shrimp with salt and pepper, then sauté until cooked.
2. In a large bowl, combine cooked quinoa, sautéed shrimp, cherry tomatoes, cucumber, red bell pepper, and avocado slices.
3. Drizzle with olive oil and lime juice, tossing gently to coat.
4. Garnish with fresh cilantro and serve with lime wedges.

## Nutritional Information: (Per Serving)
- Calories: 380
- Protein: 30g

- Carbohydrates: 30g
- Fat: 15g
- Fiber: 6g

# Caprese Sandwich with Whole Grain Bread

**Intro:** Savor the classic Italian flavors with this delightful Caprese Sandwich. Layers of fresh tomatoes, mozzarella cheese, and basil are nestled between whole grain bread, creating a simple yet delicious meal.

**Total Prep Time:** 10 minutes

**Ingredients:**
- Whole grain bread slices
- Fresh tomatoes, sliced
- Fresh mozzarella cheese, sliced
- Fresh basil leaves
- Balsamic glaze
- Olive oil
- Salt and pepper to taste

**Instructions:**
1. Drizzle olive oil on whole grain bread slices.
2. Layer fresh tomato slices, mozzarella slices, and basil leaves on the bread.
3. Drizzle with balsamic glaze.
4. Season with salt and pepper to taste.
5. Top with another slice of bread to make a sandwich.
6. Cut in half if desired and enjoy this refreshing Caprese Sandwich.

**Nutritional Information:** (Per Serving)
- Calories: 350

- Protein: 15g
- Carbohydrates: 40g
- Fat: 15g
- Fiber: 8g

# Broccoli and Cheddar Quiche

**Intro:** Indulge in a savory and cheesy delight with this Broccoli and Cheddar Quiche. The buttery crust holds a rich and creamy filling packed with broccoli and sharp cheddar cheese, making it a perfect brunch or dinner option.

**Total Prep Time:** 1 hour

**Ingredients:**
- Pie crust (store-bought or homemade)
- 2 cups broccoli florets, blanched
- 1 cup sharp cheddar cheese, shredded
- 4 large eggs
- 1 cup milk
- 1/2 teaspoon salt
- 1/4 teaspoon black pepper
- 1/4 teaspoon nutmeg (optional)

**Instructions:**
1. Preheat the oven to 375°F (190°C).
2. Line a pie dish with the pie crust.
3. Spread blanched broccoli florets and shredded cheddar cheese over the crust.
4. In a bowl, whisk together eggs, milk, salt, pepper, and nutmeg.
5. Pour the egg mixture over the broccoli and cheese.
6. Bake for 40-45 minutes or until the quiche is set and golden brown.

7. Allow it to cool for a few minutes before slicing.
8. Serve warm and enjoy this comforting Broccoli and Cheddar Quiche.

**Nutritional Information:** (Per Serving)
- Calories: 300
- Protein: 14g
- Carbohydrates: 20g
- Fat: 18g
- Fiber: 2g

# Tuna Salad Lettuce Wraps

**Intro:** Embrace a lighter meal with these Tuna Salad Lettuce Wraps. The combination of tuna, crunchy vegetables, and a zesty dressing is wrapped in crisp lettuce leaves, creating a refreshing and low-carb option.
**Total Prep Time:** 15 minutes

**Ingredients:**
- 2 cans (5 oz each) tuna, drained
- 1/4 cup mayonnaise
- 1 tablespoon Dijon mustard
- 1 celery stalk, finely chopped
- 1/4 red onion, finely chopped
- Salt and pepper to taste
- Lettuce leaves for wrapping
- Sliced cherry tomatoes for garnish
- Fresh parsley for garnish

**Instructions:**
1. In a bowl, mix together tuna, mayonnaise, Dijon mustard, celery, red onion, salt, and pepper.
2. Spoon the tuna salad onto lettuce leaves.

3. Garnish with sliced cherry tomatoes and fresh parsley.
4. Wrap the lettuce around the filling to create wraps.
5. Serve chilled and enjoy these light and flavorful Tuna Salad Lettuce Wraps.

**Nutritional Information:** (Per Serving, 2 wraps)
- Calories: 250
- Protein: 20g
- Carbohydrates: 5g
- Fat: 15g
- Fiber: 1g

# Cauliflower and Chickpea Curry

**Intro:** Dive into the aromatic spices of this Cauliflower and Chickpea Curry. The tender cauliflower and protein-packed chickpeas are simmered in a flavorful curry sauce, creating a wholesome and satisfying vegetarian dish.
**Total Prep Time:** 40 minutes

**Ingredients:**
- 1 cauliflower, cut into florets
- 1 can (15 oz) chickpeas, drained and rinsed
- 1 onion, finely chopped
- 2 cloves garlic, minced
- 1 tablespoon ginger, grated
- 1 can (14 oz) diced tomatoes
- 1 can (14 oz) coconut milk
- 2 tablespoons curry powder
- 1 teaspoon cumin
- 1 teaspoon turmeric
- 1/2 teaspoon cayenne pepper (adjust to taste)
- Salt and pepper to taste

- Fresh cilantro for garnish
- Cooked basmati rice for serving

**Instructions:**
1. In a large pan, sauté chopped onion until softened.
2. Add minced garlic and grated ginger, cook for an additional minute.
3. Stir in curry powder, cumin, turmeric, and cayenne pepper.
4. Add cauliflower florets, chickpeas, diced tomatoes, and coconut milk. Season with salt and pepper.
5. Simmer until the cauliflower is tender and the curry has thickened.
6. Garnish with fresh cilantro and serve over cooked basmati rice.

**Nutritional Information:** (Per Serving)
- Calories: 350
- Protein: 12g
- Carbohydrates: 30g
- Fat: 22g
- Fiber: 8g

## Roasted Sweet Potato and Kale Salad

**Intro:** Elevate your salad game with this Roasted Sweet Potato and Kale Salad. The combination of sweet roasted sweet potatoes, hearty kale, and a zesty vinaigrette creates a nutritious and flavorful dish.
**Total Prep Time:** 30 minutes

**Ingredients:**
- 2 sweet potatoes, peeled and diced
- 4 cups kale, stems removed and chopped

- 1/4 cup olive oil
- 1 tablespoon balsamic vinegar
- 1 teaspoon honey
- Salt and pepper to taste
- 1/4 cup feta cheese, crumbled
- 1/4 cup pecans, toasted

## Instructions:
1. Preheat the oven to 400°F (200°C).
2. Toss diced sweet potatoes with olive oil, salt, and pepper. Roast until tender.
3. Massage kale with olive oil, balsamic vinegar, honey, salt, and pepper.
4. Combine roasted sweet potatoes with kale.
5. Top with crumbled feta and toasted pecans.
6. Serve warm and enjoy this Roasted Sweet Potato and Kale Salad.

## Nutritional Information: (Per Serving)
- Calories: 300
- Protein: 5g
- Carbohydrates: 30g
- Fat: 18g
- Fiber: 6g

# Turkey and Vegetable Stir-Fry

**Intro:** Whip up a quick and healthy dinner with this Turkey and Vegetable Stir-Fry. Lean ground turkey, colorful vegetables, and a savory stir-fry sauce come together in a delicious and nutritious meal.
**Total Prep Time:** 20 minutes

### Ingredients:
- 1 lb lean ground turkey
- 2 cups broccoli florets
- 1 bell pepper, thinly sliced
- 1 carrot, julienned
- 1 zucchini, sliced
- 3 tablespoons soy sauce
- 1 tablespoon hoisin sauce
- 1 tablespoon sesame oil
- 1 tablespoon ginger, grated
- 2 cloves garlic, minced
- Green onions for garnish
- Sesame seeds for garnish

### Instructions:
1. In a wok or large skillet, brown ground turkey over medium heat.
2. Add broccoli, bell pepper, carrot, and zucchini. Stir-fry until vegetables are tender-crisp.
3. In a small bowl, mix soy sauce, hoisin sauce, sesame oil, ginger, and garlic.
4. Pour the sauce over the turkey and vegetables, tossing to coat evenly.
5. Cook for an additional 2-3 minutes until heated through.
6. Garnish with green onions and sesame seeds.
7. Serve hot and enjoy this Turkey and Vegetable Stir-Fry.

### Nutritional Information: (Per Serving)
- Calories: 320
- Protein: 25g
- Carbohydrates: 15g
- Fat: 18g

- Fiber: 5g

# Quinoa and Black-Eyed Pea Salad

**Intro:** Embrace a protein-packed salad with this Quinoa and Black-Eyed Pea Salad. The combination of quinoa, black-eyed peas, and a vibrant medley of vegetables makes for a hearty and nutritious dish.
**Total Prep Time:** 25 minutes

**Ingredients:**
- 1 cup quinoa, cooked
- 1 can (15 oz) black-eyed peas, drained and rinsed
- 1 cup cherry tomatoes, halved
- 1 cucumber, diced
- 1/4 cup red onion, finely chopped
- 1/4 cup fresh cilantro, chopped
- Juice of 1 lemon
- 2 tablespoons olive oil
- Salt and pepper to taste
- Feta cheese for garnish (optional)

**Instructions:**
1. In a large bowl, combine cooked quinoa, black-eyed peas, cherry tomatoes, cucumber, red onion, and cilantro.
2. In a small bowl, whisk together lemon juice, olive oil, salt, and pepper.
3. Pour the dressing over the salad and toss to combine.
4. Garnish with crumbled feta cheese if desired.
5. Serve chilled and enjoy this Quinoa and Black-Eyed Pea Salad.

**Nutritional Information:** (Per Serving)
- Calories: 280
- Protein: 9g
- Carbohydrates: 40g
- Fat: 10g
- Fiber: 8g

## Pesto Zoodle Bowl with Cherry Tomatoes

**Intro:** Explore a lighter alternative to pasta with this Pesto Zoodle Bowl. Spiralized zucchini noodles are tossed in a vibrant pesto sauce and topped with cherry tomatoes for a fresh and flavorful experience.

**Total Prep Time:** 15 minutes

### Ingredients:
- 4 medium zucchini, spiralized
- 1 cup cherry tomatoes, halved
- 1/2 cup basil pesto
- Parmesan cheese for garnish
- Pine nuts for garnish (optional)
- Salt and pepper to taste

### Instructions:
1. Spiralize zucchini to create "zoodles."
2. In a large bowl, toss zoodles with cherry tomatoes and basil pesto.
3. Season with salt and pepper to taste.
4. Garnish with Parmesan cheese and pine nuts if desired.
5. Serve immediately, savoring the freshness of this Pesto Zoodle Bowl.

**Nutritional Information:** (Per Serving)

- Calories: 180
- Protein: 5g
- Carbohydrates: 10g
- Fat: 15g
- Fiber: 3g

# Mexican Quinoa Bowl with Avocado

**Intro:** Spice up your mealtime with this Mexican Quinoa Bowl featuring the goodness of quinoa, black beans, corn, and avocado. Topped with a zesty lime dressing, it's a satisfying and flavorful dish.

**Total Prep Time:** 30 minutes

**Ingredients:**

- 1 cup quinoa, cooked
- 1 can (15 oz) black beans, drained and rinsed
- 1 cup corn kernels (fresh or frozen)
- 1 avocado, sliced
- Cherry tomatoes, halved
- Red onion, finely chopped
- Fresh cilantro, chopped
- Lime dressing: Juice of 2 limes, 2 tablespoons olive oil, 1 teaspoon cumin, salt and pepper to taste

**Instructions:**

1. In a bowl, combine cooked quinoa, black beans, corn, avocado, cherry tomatoes, and red onion.
2. In a small jar, shake together lime juice, olive oil, cumin, salt, and pepper to create the dressing.
3. Drizzle the lime dressing over the quinoa bowl.
4. Garnish with fresh cilantro.

5. Toss gently and serve this vibrant Mexican Quinoa Bowl.

**Nutritional Information:** (Per Serving)
- Calories: 350
- Protein: 12g
- Carbohydrates: 45g
- Fat: 15g
- Fiber: 10g

# Mexican Quinoa Bowl with Avocado

**Intro:** Dive into the vibrant flavors of this Mexican Quinoa Bowl with Avocado. Packed with protein-rich quinoa, black beans, corn, and creamy avocado, this bowl is a nutritious and satisfying meal. Topped with a zesty lime dressing, it's a fiesta for your taste buds.

**Total Prep Time:** 30 minutes

**Ingredients:**
- 1 cup quinoa, cooked
- 1 can (15 oz) black beans, drained and rinsed
- 1 cup corn kernels (fresh or frozen)
- 1 avocado, sliced
- Cherry tomatoes, halved
- Red onion, finely chopped
- Fresh cilantro, chopped
- Lime dressing: Juice of 2 limes, 2 tablespoons olive oil, 1 teaspoon cumin, salt and pepper to taste

**Instructions:**
1. In a bowl, combine cooked quinoa, black beans, corn, avocado, cherry tomatoes, and red onion.

2. In a small jar, shake together lime juice, olive oil, cumin, salt, and pepper to create the dressing.
3. Drizzle the lime dressing over the quinoa bowl.
4. Garnish with fresh cilantro.
5. Toss gently and serve this vibrant Mexican Quinoa Bowl.

**Nutritional Information:** (Per Serving)
- Calories: 350
- Protein: 12g
- Carbohydrates: 45g
- Fat: 15g
- Fiber: 10g

# Chicken and Vegetable Skewers with Tzatziki Sauce

**Intro:** Elevate your grilling game with these Chicken and Vegetable Skewers paired with refreshing Tzatziki Sauce. The marinated chicken, colorful vegetables, and tangy tzatziki create a delicious and wholesome dish perfect for a summer barbecue.

**Total Prep Time:** 25 minutes (plus marination time)

**Ingredients:**
- 1 lb chicken breast, cut into chunks
- Bell peppers, cherry tomatoes, red onion (for skewering)
- Olive oil
- 2 teaspoons dried oregano
- 1 teaspoon garlic powder
- Salt and pepper to taste
- Wooden or metal skewers

**Tzatziki Sauce:**
- 1 cup Greek yogurt
- 1/2 cucumber, finely diced
- 2 tablespoons fresh dill, chopped
- 1 clove garlic, minced
- Juice of 1 lemon
- Salt and pepper to taste

**Instructions:**
1. In a bowl, combine chicken chunks with olive oil, dried oregano, garlic powder, salt, and pepper. Marinate for at least 30 minutes.
2. Thread marinated chicken, bell peppers, cherry tomatoes, and red onion onto skewers.
3. Grill skewers until chicken is fully cooked and vegetables are charred.
4. For the Tzatziki Sauce, mix together Greek yogurt, diced cucumber, fresh dill, minced garlic, lemon juice, salt, and pepper.
5. Serve Chicken and Vegetable Skewers with a side of Tzatziki Sauce.

**Nutritional Information:** (Per Serving)
- Calories: 300
- Protein: 30g
- Carbohydrates: 15g
- Fat: 15g
- Fiber: 3g

## Mediterranean Chickpea Salad

**Intro:** Immerse yourself in the flavors of the Mediterranean with this refreshing Chickpea Salad. Packed with chickpeas, cherry tomatoes, cucumber, olives, and feta cheese, it's tossed in a lemon-oregano dressing for a light and zesty experience.

**Total Prep Time:** 20 minutes

## Ingredients:
- 2 cans (15 oz each) chickpeas, drained and rinsed
- 1 cup cherry tomatoes, halved
- 1 cucumber, diced
- 1/2 cup Kalamata olives, sliced
- 1/2 cup feta cheese, crumbled
- 1/4 cup red onion, finely chopped
- Fresh parsley, chopped
- Dressing: Juice of 2 lemons, 1/4 cup olive oil, 1 teaspoon dried oregano, salt and pepper to taste

## Instructions:
1. In a large bowl, combine chickpeas, cherry tomatoes, cucumber, olives, feta cheese, and red onion.
2. In a small bowl, whisk together lemon juice, olive oil, dried oregano, salt, and pepper to create the dressing.
3. Pour the dressing over the salad and toss gently.
4. Garnish with fresh parsley.
5. Serve chilled and enjoy this Mediterranean Chickpea Salad.

## Nutritional Information: (Per Serving)
- Calories: 320
- Protein: 12g
- Carbohydrates: 40g
- Fat: 15g
- Fiber: 10g

# Salmon and Asparagus Foil Pack

**Intro:** Simplify dinner with this easy and flavorful Salmon and Asparagus Foil Pack. The combination of salmon fillets, fresh asparagus, and a lemon-dill marinade creates a delicious and fuss-free meal. Perfect for a quick weeknight dinner or a weekend barbecue.

**Total Prep Time:** 30 minutes

## Ingredients:
- 4 salmon fillets
- 1 bunch asparagus, trimmed
- 1 lemon, thinly sliced
- Fresh dill, chopped
- 2 tablespoons olive oil
- Salt and pepper to taste

## Instructions:
1. Preheat the oven to 400°F (200°C).
2. Lay out four sheets of aluminum foil.
3. Place a salmon fillet on each foil sheet, surrounded by asparagus spears.
4. Drizzle olive oil over each salmon fillet and asparagus.
5. Season with salt, pepper, and fresh dill.
6. Top each fillet with lemon slices.
7. Seal the foil packs tightly and place them on a baking sheet.
8. Bake for 15-20 minutes or until salmon is cooked through.
9. Serve hot, unwrapping the foil to reveal the delicious Salmon and Asparagus Foil Pack.

**Nutritional Information:** (Per Serving)
- Calories: 350
- Protein: 30g
- Carbohydrates: 10g
- Fat: 22g
- Fiber: 4g

## Asian-Inspired Turkey Lettuce Wraps

**Intro:** Experience the vibrant flavors of Asia with these Asian-Inspired Turkey Lettuce Wraps. Ground turkey is cooked with a savory blend of Asian-inspired seasonings and nestled in crisp lettuce leaves, creating a light and delicious meal.

**Total Prep Time:** 25 minutes

**Ingredients:**
- 1 lb ground turkey
- 1 tablespoon sesame oil
- 2 cloves garlic, minced
- 1 tablespoon ginger, grated
- 1/4 cup soy sauce
- 2 tablespoons hoisin sauce
- 1 tablespoon rice vinegar
- 1 teaspoon Sriracha (adjust to taste)
- 1 cup water chestnuts, chopped
- 1/4 cup green onions, sliced
- Lettuce leaves for wrapping

**Instructions:**
1. In a skillet, heat sesame oil over medium heat.
2. Add ground turkey and cook until browned.
3. Add minced garlic and grated ginger, cooking for an additional minute.

4. Stir in soy sauce, hoisin sauce, rice vinegar, and Sriracha.
5. Add chopped water chestnuts and sliced green onions, mixing well.
6. Simmer for 5-7 minutes until flavors meld.
7. Spoon the turkey mixture onto lettuce leaves.
8. Serve hot and enjoy these Asian-Inspired Turkey Lettuce Wraps.

**Nutritional Information:** (Per Serving, 2 wraps)
- Calories: 280
- Protein: 25g
- Carbohydrates: 10g
- Fat: 15g
- Fiber: 3g

## Minestrone Soup with Whole Wheat Pasta

**Intro:** Warm up with a comforting bowl of Minestrone Soup featuring wholesome whole wheat pasta. This hearty soup is loaded with vegetables, beans, and a flavorful broth, making it a nourishing and satisfying meal.
**Total Prep Time:** 40 minutes

**Ingredients:**
- 1 cup whole wheat pasta, cooked
- 1 onion, diced
- 2 carrots, diced
- 2 celery stalks, diced
- 3 cloves garlic, minced
- 1 can (15 oz) diced tomatoes
- 1 can (15 oz) kidney beans, drained and rinsed
- 4 cups vegetable broth
- 1 teaspoon dried oregano

- 1 teaspoon dried basil
- Salt and pepper to taste
- Fresh parsley for garnish
- Grated Parmesan cheese for serving

## Instructions:
1. In a large pot, sauté diced onion, carrots, and celery until softened.
2. Add minced garlic and cook for an additional minute.
3. Stir in diced tomatoes, kidney beans, vegetable broth, oregano, basil, salt, and pepper.
4. Bring the soup to a boil, then reduce heat and simmer for 20-25 minutes.
5. Add cooked whole wheat pasta and simmer for an additional 5 minutes.
6. Adjust seasoning as needed.
7. Garnish with fresh parsley and serve hot with grated Parmesan cheese.

## Nutritional Information: (Per Serving)
- Calories: 300
- Protein: 12g
- Carbohydrates: 50g
- Fat: 4g
- Fiber: 10g

# Egg Salad Lettuce Wraps

**Intro:** Enjoy a light and protein-packed lunch with these Egg Salad Lettuce Wraps. Creamy egg salad is nestled in crisp lettuce leaves, creating a refreshing and satisfying dish.

**Total Prep Time:** 15 minutes

**Ingredients:**
- 6 hard-boiled eggs, chopped
- 1/4 cup mayonnaise
- 1 tablespoon Dijon mustard
- 1/4 cup celery, finely chopped
- 2 tablespoons red onion, finely chopped
- Salt and pepper to taste
- Lettuce leaves for wrapping

**Instructions:**
1. In a bowl, mix together chopped hard-boiled eggs, mayonnaise, Dijon mustard, celery, red onion, salt, and pepper.
2. Spoon the egg salad onto lettuce leaves.
3. Serve chilled and enjoy these Egg Salad Lettuce Wraps.

**Nutritional Information:** (Per Serving, 2 wraps)
- Calories: 250
- Protein: 15g
- Carbohydrates: 5g
- Fat: 18g
- Fiber: 1g

## Spicy Tofu and Vegetable Stir-Fry

**Intro:** Add a kick to your dinner routine with this Spicy Tofu and Vegetable Stir-Fry. Cubes of tofu, colorful vegetables, and a spicy sauce come together in a flavorful and satisfying stir-fry.

**Total Prep Time:** 30 minutes

**Ingredients:**
- 1 block firm tofu, pressed and cubed

- 2 tablespoons soy sauce
- 1 tablespoon hoisin sauce
- 1 tablespoon Sriracha (adjust to taste)
- 1 tablespoon sesame oil
- 1 tablespoon vegetable oil
- 2 bell peppers, sliced
- 1 cup broccoli florets
- 1 carrot, julienned
- 2 cloves garlic, minced
- 1 tablespoon ginger, grated
- Green onions for garnish
- Sesame seeds for garnish
- Cooked brown rice for serving

## Instructions:
1. In a bowl, marinate cubed tofu in soy sauce, hoisin sauce, and Sriracha.
2. Heat vegetable oil and sesame oil in a wok or skillet.
3. Add marinated tofu and cook until golden brown.
4. Stir in sliced bell peppers, broccoli florets, julienned carrot, minced garlic, and grated ginger.
5. Cook until vegetables are tender-crisp.
6. Garnish with green onions and sesame seeds.
7. Serve over cooked brown rice and enjoy this Spicy Tofu and Vegetable Stir-Fry.

## Nutritional Information: (Per Serving)
- Calories: 350
- Protein: 15g
- Carbohydrates: 30g
- Fat: 20g
- Fiber: 6g

# Cucumber and Avocado Sushi Bowl

**Intro:** Experience the flavors of sushi without the rolling with this Cucumber and Avocado Sushi Bowl. Fresh cucumber, creamy avocado, and sushi rice are drizzled with a soy-based dressing, creating a deconstructed sushi experience.

**Total Prep Time:** 20 minutes

## Ingredients:
- 2 cups sushi rice, cooked and seasoned with rice vinegar
- 1 cucumber, julienned
- 1 avocado, sliced
- 1 nori sheet, shredded
- 2 tablespoons soy sauce
- 1 tablespoon rice vinegar
- 1 tablespoon sesame oil
- 1 teaspoon sugar
- Sesame seeds for garnish
- Pickled ginger and wasabi for serving (optional)

## Instructions:
1. In a bowl, assemble sushi rice, julienned cucumber, sliced avocado, and shredded nori.
2. In a separate bowl, whisk together soy sauce, rice vinegar, sesame oil, and sugar to create the dressing.
3. Drizzle the dressing over the sushi bowl.
4. Garnish with sesame seeds.
5. Serve with pickled ginger and wasabi if desired.
6. Enjoy this Cucumber and Avocado Sushi Bowl.

**Nutritional Information:** (Per Serving)
- Calories: 400
- Protein: 5g
- Carbohydrates: 70g
- Fat: 12g
- Fiber: 5g

# Baked Salmon with Lemon and Dill

**Intro:** Elevate your dinner with this Baked Salmon with Lemon and Dill. The combination of succulent salmon fillets, zesty lemon, and aromatic dill creates a simple yet elegant dish. Perfect for a healthy and flavorful meal.
**Total Prep Time:** 25 minutes

**Ingredients:**
- 4 salmon fillets
- 2 lemons, thinly sliced
- 2 tablespoons fresh dill, chopped
- 2 tablespoons olive oil
- Salt and pepper to taste

**Instructions:**
1. Preheat the oven to 375°F (190°C).
2. Place salmon fillets on a baking sheet lined with parchment paper.
3. Season with salt and pepper.
4. Lay lemon slices on top of each fillet.
5. Drizzle with olive oil and sprinkle chopped dill.
6. Bake for 15-18 minutes or until the salmon is cooked through.
7. Serve hot and enjoy this Baked Salmon with Lemon and Dill.

**Nutritional Information:** (Per Serving)
- Calories: 300
- Protein: 30g
- Carbohydrates: 2g
- Fat: 20g
- Fiber: 1g

# Grilled Chicken with Quinoa Pilaf

**Intro:** Delight your taste buds with this Grilled Chicken with Quinoa Pilaf. Tender grilled chicken is served alongside a flavorful quinoa pilaf, creating a protein-packed and satisfying meal.
**Total Prep Time:** 30 minutes

**Ingredients:**
- 4 chicken breasts, boneless and skinless
- 1 cup quinoa, cooked
- 1 cup cherry tomatoes, halved
- 1 cucumber, diced
- 1/4 cup red onion, finely chopped
- 2 tablespoons feta cheese, crumbled
- 2 tablespoons olive oil
- Juice of 1 lemon
- Fresh parsley for garnish
- Salt and pepper to taste

**Instructions:**
1. Season chicken breasts with salt and pepper.
2. Grill chicken until fully cooked.
3. In a bowl, combine cooked quinoa, cherry tomatoes, cucumber, red onion, and feta cheese.
4. Drizzle olive oil and lemon juice over the quinoa pilaf.

5. Slice grilled chicken and serve over the quinoa mixture.
6. Garnish with fresh parsley.
7. Serve warm and enjoy Grilled Chicken with Quinoa Pilaf.

**Nutritional Information:** (Per Serving)
- Calories: 400
- Protein: 35g
- Carbohydrates: 30g
- Fat: 15g
- Fiber: 4g

# Vegetable and Lentil Stew

**Intro:** Embrace the wholesome goodness of this Vegetable and Lentil Stew. Packed with nutritious vegetables and protein-rich lentils, this hearty stew is a comforting and satisfying choice for a wholesome meal.

**Total Prep Time:** 40 minutes

**Ingredients:**
- 1 cup dry green lentils, rinsed
- 4 cups vegetable broth
- 2 carrots, diced
- 2 celery stalks, diced
- 1 onion, chopped
- 3 cloves garlic, minced
- 1 can (15 oz) diced tomatoes
- 1 cup green beans, chopped
- 1 cup kale, chopped
- 1 teaspoon dried thyme
- 1 teaspoon cumin
- Salt and pepper to taste

- Fresh parsley for garnish

## Instructions:
1. In a large pot, combine green lentils and vegetable broth. Bring to a boil.
2. Add carrots, celery, onion, and garlic to the pot.
3. Stir in diced tomatoes, green beans, kale, thyme, cumin, salt, and pepper.
4. Simmer for 25-30 minutes or until lentils are tender.
5. Adjust seasoning as needed.
6. Garnish with fresh parsley.
7. Serve hot and enjoy this Vegetable and Lentil Stew.

## Nutritional Information: (Per Serving)
- Calories: 300
- Protein: 18g
- Carbohydrates: 50g
- Fat: 2g
- Fiber: 15g

# Turkey and Sweet Potato Chili

**Intro:** Warm up with the comforting flavors of Turkey and Sweet Potato Chili. Lean ground turkey, sweet potatoes, and a medley of spices come together in a hearty and nutritious chili that's perfect for chilly evenings.

**Total Prep Time:** 45 minutes

## Ingredients:
- 1 lb lean ground turkey
- 2 sweet potatoes, peeled and diced
- 1 onion, chopped
- 3 cloves garlic, minced

- 1 can (15 oz) black beans, drained and rinsed
- 1 can (15 oz) kidney beans, drained and rinsed
- 1 can (15 oz) diced tomatoes
- 2 cups chicken broth
- 2 tablespoons chili powder
- 1 teaspoon cumin
- 1 teaspoon paprika
- Salt and pepper to taste
- Green onions and shredded cheddar for garnish

**Instructions:**
1. In a large pot, brown ground turkey over medium heat.
2. Add chopped sweet potatoes, onion, and garlic. Cook until vegetables are softened.
3. Stir in black beans, kidney beans, diced tomatoes, chicken broth, chili powder, cumin, paprika, salt, and pepper.
4. Bring to a simmer and let it cook for 30 minutes, allowing flavors to meld.
5. Adjust seasoning as needed.
6. Serve hot, garnished with green onions and shredded cheddar.

**Nutritional Information:** (Per Serving)
- Calories: 350
- Protein: 25g
- Carbohydrates: 40g
- Fat: 10g
- Fiber: 12g

# Eggplant Parmesan with Whole Wheat Pasta

**Intro:** Indulge in a healthier twist on a classic Italian dish with this Eggplant Parmesan with Whole Wheat Pasta. Crispy baked eggplant slices are layered with marinara sauce and melted mozzarella, served over whole wheat pasta for a satisfying and flavorful meal.

**Total Prep Time:** 1 hour

## Ingredients:
- 1 large eggplant, sliced
- 1 cup whole wheat pasta, cooked
- 2 cups marinara sauce
- 1 cup mozzarella cheese, shredded
- 1/2 cup Parmesan cheese, grated
- Fresh basil for garnish
- Olive oil for brushing
- Salt and pepper to taste

## Instructions:
1. Preheat the oven to 400°F (200°C).
2. Brush eggplant slices with olive oil and season with salt and pepper.
3. Bake for 20-25 minutes or until golden brown.
4. In a baking dish, layer cooked whole wheat pasta, marinara sauce, baked eggplant slices, mozzarella, and Parmesan cheese.
5. Repeat the layers.
6. Bake for an additional 20 minutes or until the cheese is melted and bubbly.
7. Garnish with fresh basil.
8. Serve hot and enjoy Eggplant Parmesan with Whole Wheat Pasta.

**Nutritional Information:** (Per Serving)
- Calories: 400
- Protein: 18g
- Carbohydrates: 45g
- Fat: 18g
- Fiber: 10g

# Teriyaki Glazed Tofu with Broccoli

**Intro:** Explore the savory-sweet goodness of Teriyaki Glazed Tofu with Broccoli. Tofu cubes are pan-seared to perfection and coated in a homemade teriyaki sauce, creating a delicious and wholesome dish.
**Total Prep Time:** 30 minutes

**Ingredients:**
- 1 block firm tofu, pressed and cubed
- 3 cups broccoli florets
- 1/4 cup low-sodium soy sauce
- 2 tablespoons mirin
- 2 tablespoons rice vinegar
- 1 tablespoon maple syrup
- 1 tablespoon cornstarch
- 1 tablespoon vegetable oil
- Sesame seeds for garnish
- Green onions for garnish
- Cooked brown rice for serving

**Instructions:**
1. In a bowl, whisk together soy sauce, mirin, rice vinegar, maple syrup, and cornstarch to create the teriyaki sauce.
2. In a pan, heat vegetable oil over medium heat.

3. Add tofu cubes and cook until golden brown on all sides.
4. Add broccoli florets to the pan and sauté until tender-crisp.
5. Pour the teriyaki sauce over tofu and broccoli, stirring to coat.
6. Cook for an additional 2-3 minutes until the sauce thickens.
7. Serve over cooked brown rice, garnished with sesame seeds and green onions.
8. Enjoy Teriyaki Glazed Tofu with Broccoli.

**Nutritional Information:** (Per Serving)
- Calories: 350
- Protein: 18g
- Carbohydrates: 40g
- Fat: 15g
- Fiber: 6g

# Quinoa-Stuffed Bell Peppers

**Intro:** Delight in a nutritious and colorful meal with these Quinoa-Stuffed Bell Peppers. Quinoa is mixed with a medley of vegetables and spices, then baked to perfection inside vibrant bell peppers.
**Total Prep Time:** 40 minutes

**Ingredients:**
- 1 cup quinoa, cooked
- 4 bell peppers, halved and seeds removed
- 1 can (15 oz) black beans, drained and rinsed
- 1 cup corn kernels (fresh or frozen)
- 1 cup cherry tomatoes, diced
- 1/2 cup red onion, finely chopped

- 1 teaspoon cumin
- 1 teaspoon chili powder
- Salt and pepper to taste
- 1 cup shredded cheddar cheese
- Fresh cilantro for garnish
- Lime wedges for serving

## Instructions:
1. Preheat the oven to 375°F (190°C).
2. In a bowl, combine cooked quinoa, black beans, corn, cherry tomatoes, red onion, cumin, chili powder, salt, and pepper.
3. Stuff each bell pepper half with the quinoa mixture.
4. Top with shredded cheddar cheese.
5. Bake for 25-30 minutes or until the peppers are tender.
6. Garnish with fresh cilantro.
7. Serve hot with lime wedges.
8. Enjoy these Quinoa-Stuffed Bell Peppers.

**Nutritional Information:** (Per Serving, 2 halves)
- Calories: 350
- Protein: 15g
- Carbohydrates: 45g
- Fat: 15g
- Fiber: 8g

# Lemon Herb Roasted Chicken

**Intro:** Indulge in the savory goodness of Lemon Herb Roasted Chicken. Juicy chicken is marinated in a flavorful blend of herbs and roasted to perfection, creating a mouthwatering and aromatic dish.

**Total Prep Time:** 1 hour and 15 minutes

**Ingredients:**
- 4 chicken thighs, bone-in and skin-on
- 1 lemon, juiced and zested
- 2 tablespoons olive oil
- 3 cloves garlic, minced
- 1 tablespoon fresh rosemary, chopped
- 1 tablespoon fresh thyme, chopped
- Salt and pepper to taste

**Instructions:**
1. Preheat the oven to 400°F (200°C).
2. In a bowl, whisk together lemon juice, lemon zest, olive oil, minced garlic, chopped rosemary, chopped thyme, salt, and pepper.
3. Place chicken thighs in a baking dish and pour the lemon herb marinade over them, ensuring they are well-coated.
4. Marinate for at least 30 minutes.
5. Roast chicken in the preheated oven for 40-45 minutes or until the skin is golden brown and the internal temperature reaches 165°F (74°C).
6. Let it rest for 10 minutes before serving.
7. Serve hot and enjoy Lemon Herb Roasted Chicken.

**Nutritional Information:** (Per Serving)
- Calories: 400
- Protein: 25g
- Carbohydrates: 2g
- Fat: 35g
- Fiber: 1g

# Shrimp and Zucchini Noodles with Pesto

**Intro:** Indulge in a light and flavorful dish with Shrimp and Zucchini Noodles with Pesto. Tender shrimp is sautéed with zucchini noodles and tossed in a vibrant pesto sauce, creating a low-carb and delicious meal.
**Total Prep Time:** 20 minutes

**Ingredients:**
- 1 lb shrimp, peeled and deveined
- 4 medium zucchinis, spiralized into noodles
- 1/2 cup cherry tomatoes, halved
- 1/4 cup pine nuts, toasted
- 1/2 cup fresh basil leaves
- 2 cloves garlic, minced
- 1/2 cup Parmesan cheese, grated
- 1/2 cup extra-virgin olive oil
- Salt and pepper to taste
- Red pepper flakes for garnish
- Lemon wedges for serving

**Instructions:**
1. In a blender, combine basil, garlic, Parmesan cheese, and pine nuts. Blend until well combined.
2. With the blender running, slowly pour in the olive oil until a smooth pesto sauce forms. Season with salt and pepper.
3. In a large skillet, sauté shrimp until pink and cooked through. Remove from the skillet and set aside.
4. In the same skillet, add zucchini noodles and cherry tomatoes. Cook until just tender.
5. Toss cooked shrimp and pesto sauce with zucchini noodles until well combined.

6. Garnish with red pepper flakes.
7. Serve hot with lemon wedges.
8. Enjoy Shrimp and Zucchini Noodles with Pesto.

**Nutritional Information:** (Per Serving)
- Calories: 350
- Protein: 25g
- Carbohydrates: 10g
- Fat: 25g
- Fiber: 3g

# Mediterranean Baked Cod

**Intro:** Transport your taste buds to the Mediterranean with this flavorful and healthy dish of Mediterranean Baked Cod. Cod fillets are baked with a medley of tomatoes, olives, and herbs, creating a light and satisfying meal.
**Total Prep Time:** 30 minutes

**Ingredients:**
- 4 cod fillets
- 1 cup cherry tomatoes, halved
- 1/2 cup Kalamata olives, pitted and sliced
- 3 tablespoons capers
- 3 tablespoons fresh parsley, chopped
- 2 tablespoons olive oil
- 2 cloves garlic, minced
- 1 teaspoon dried oregano
- Salt and pepper to taste
- Lemon wedges for serving

**Instructions:**
1. Preheat the oven to 400°F (200°C).
2. In a bowl, combine cherry tomatoes, olives, capers, parsley, olive oil, minced garlic, oregano, salt, and pepper.
3. Place cod fillets in a baking dish and top with the Mediterranean mixture.
4. Bake for 15-20 minutes or until the cod is opaque and flakes easily.
5. Garnish with additional fresh parsley.
6. Serve hot with lemon wedges.
7. Enjoy Mediterranean Baked Cod.

**Nutritional Information:** (Per Serving)
- Calories: 250
- Protein: 30g
- Carbohydrates: 5g
- Fat: 12g
- Fiber: 2g

# Spaghetti Squash with Tomato and Basil Sauce

**Intro:** Embrace a lighter alternative to traditional pasta with Spaghetti Squash with Tomato and Basil Sauce. Roasted spaghetti squash strands are tossed with a fresh tomato and basil sauce, creating a low-carb and flavorful dish.

**Total Prep Time:** 45 minutes

**Ingredients:**
- 1 large spaghetti squash, halved and seeds removed
- 2 cups cherry tomatoes, halved
- 1/4 cup fresh basil, chopped

- 2 cloves garlic, minced
- 2 tablespoons olive oil
- Salt and pepper to taste
- Grated Parmesan cheese for serving

## Instructions:
1. Preheat the oven to 400°F (200°C).
2. Brush the cut sides of the spaghetti squash with olive oil and season with salt and pepper.
3. Place the squash, cut side down, on a baking sheet.
4. Roast for 35-40 minutes or until the squash is tender and the strands easily separate with a fork.
5. In a pan, sauté cherry tomatoes and minced garlic in olive oil until tomatoes are softened.
6. Using a fork, scrape the spaghetti squash strands into a bowl.
7. Toss the squash with the tomato and basil sauce.
8. Serve hot, garnished with fresh basil and grated Parmesan cheese.
9. Enjoy Spaghetti Squash with Tomato and Basil Sauce.

**Nutritional Information:** (Per Serving)
- Calories: 200
- Protein: 3g
- Carbohydrates: 20g
- Fat: 12g
- Fiber: 4g

# Black Bean and Vegetable Enchiladas

**Intro:** Dive into the flavors of Mexico with these Black Bean and Vegetable Enchiladas. Flour tortillas are filled with a savory mixture of black beans, vegetables, and cheese, then baked to perfection and topped with a zesty enchilada sauce.

**Total Prep Time:** 40 minutes

## Ingredients:
- 1 can (15 oz) black beans, drained and rinsed
- 1 cup corn kernels (fresh or frozen)
- 1 bell pepper, diced
- 1 zucchini, diced
- 1 onion, chopped
- 2 cloves garlic, minced
- 1 teaspoon cumin
- 1 teaspoon chili powder
- Salt and pepper to taste
- 8 small flour tortillas
- 2 cups shredded Mexican cheese blend
- 1 can (15 oz) red enchilada sauce
- Fresh cilantro for garnish
- Avocado slices for serving

## Instructions:
1. Preheat the oven to 375°F (190°C).
2. In a pan, sauté onion and garlic until softened.
3. Add bell pepper, zucchini, cumin, chili powder, salt, and pepper. Cook until vegetables are tender.
4. Stir in black beans and corn. Cook for an additional 2-3 minutes.
5. In a separate pan, warm tortillas.
6. Fill each tortilla with the vegetable and bean mixture, then roll and place seam-side down in a baking dish.
7. Pour enchilada sauce over the rolled tortillas and top with shredded cheese.

8. Bake for 20-25 minutes or until the cheese is melted and bubbly.
9. Garnish with fresh cilantro and serve with avocado slices.
10. Enjoy Black Bean and Vegetable Enchiladas.

**Nutritional Information:** (Per Serving, 2 enchiladas)
- Calories: 400
- Protein: 15g
- Carbohydrates: 45g
- Fat: 18g
- Fiber: 8g

# Chicken and Vegetable Curry

**Intro:** Transport your taste buds to the vibrant flavors of India with Chicken and Vegetable Curry. Tender chicken, mixed vegetables, and aromatic spices come together in a rich and flavorful curry that's perfect served over rice or with naan.

**Total Prep Time:** 45 minutes

**Ingredients:**
- 1 lb boneless, skinless chicken thighs, cut into cubes
- 1 onion, finely chopped
- 2 cloves garlic, minced
- 1 tablespoon ginger, grated
- 1 can (14 oz) diced tomatoes
- 1 cup mixed vegetables (peas, carrots, bell peppers)
- 1/2 cup coconut milk
- 2 tablespoons curry powder
- 1 teaspoon turmeric
- 1 teaspoon cumin
- Salt and pepper to taste

- Fresh cilantro for garnish
- Cooked rice or naan for serving

**Instructions:**
1. In a pot, sauté onion, garlic, and ginger until fragrant.
2. Add chicken cubes and cook until browned.
3. Stir in diced tomatoes, mixed vegetables, coconut milk, curry powder, turmeric, cumin, salt, and pepper.
4. Simmer for 25-30 minutes or until chicken is cooked through and flavors meld.
5. Adjust seasoning as needed.
6. Serve over rice or with naan.
7. Garnish with fresh cilantro.
8. Enjoy Chicken and Vegetable Curry.

**Nutritional Information:** (Per Serving)
- Calories: 450
- Protein: 30g
- Carbohydrates: 20g
- Fat: 25g
- Fiber: 5g

# Roasted Brussels Sprouts and Quinoa Bowl

**Intro:** Elevate your lunch or dinner with the Roasted Brussels Sprouts and Quinoa Bowl. Nutrient-rich quinoa is topped with roasted Brussels sprouts, chickpeas, and a drizzle of balsamic glaze, creating a wholesome and satisfying dish.

**Total Prep Time:** 30 minutes

## Ingredients:
- 1 cup quinoa, cooked
- 1 lb Brussels sprouts, halved
- 1 can (15 oz) chickpeas, drained and rinsed
- 2 tablespoons olive oil
- Salt and pepper to taste
- Balsamic glaze for drizzling
- Fresh parsley for garnish
- Lemon wedges for serving

## Instructions:
1. Preheat the oven to 400°F (200°C).
2. Toss Brussels sprouts and chickpeas with olive oil, salt, and pepper.
3. Roast in the oven for 20-25 minutes or until Brussels sprouts are golden brown and chickpeas are crispy.
4. In a bowl, assemble cooked quinoa, roasted Brussels sprouts, and chickpeas.
5. Drizzle with balsamic glaze.
6. Garnish with fresh parsley and serve with lemon wedges.
7. Enjoy the Roasted Brussels Sprouts and Quinoa Bowl.

## Nutritional Information: (Per Serving)
- Calories: 350
- Protein: 15g
- Carbohydrates: 50g
- Fat: 10g
- Fiber: 10g

# Cauliflower Crust Margherita Pizza

**Intro:** Satisfy your pizza cravings with a healthier twist – Cauliflower Crust Margherita Pizza. A cauliflower crust is topped with fresh tomatoes, mozzarella, and basil, creating a delicious and guilt-free pizza experience.
**Total Prep Time:** 45 minutes

## Ingredients:
- 1 medium cauliflower, riced
- 1/2 cup mozzarella cheese, shredded
- 1/4 cup Parmesan cheese, grated
- 1 egg
- 1 teaspoon dried oregano
- 1/2 teaspoon garlic powder
- Salt and pepper to taste
- 1/2 cup tomato sauce
- 1 cup fresh mozzarella, sliced
- 2-3 tomatoes, sliced
- Fresh basil leaves for garnish
- Red pepper flakes (optional)

## Instructions:
1. Preheat the oven to 425°F (220°C).
2. Place riced cauliflower in a microwave-safe bowl and microwave for 5 minutes. Let it cool.
3. Mix cauliflower with mozzarella cheese, Parmesan cheese, egg, oregano, garlic powder, salt, and pepper.
4. Spread the cauliflower mixture on a parchment-lined baking sheet, shaping it into a round crust.
5. Bake for 20-25 minutes or until the crust is golden brown.

6. Remove from the oven and spread tomato sauce over the crust.
7. Arrange fresh mozzarella and tomato slices on top.
8. Bake for an additional 10-15 minutes or until the cheese is melted and bubbly.
9. Garnish with fresh basil and red pepper flakes if desired.
10. Slice and enjoy Cauliflower Crust Margherita Pizza.

**Nutritional Information:** (Per Serving)
- Calories: 250
- Protein: 15g
- Carbohydrates: 15g
- Fat: 15g
- Fiber: 5g

# Beef and Vegetable Stir-Fry

**Intro:** Stir up a quick and flavorful dinner with Beef and Vegetable Stir-Fry. Tender strips of beef are wok-tossed with colorful vegetables in a savory soy-based sauce, creating a delicious and nutritious meal in minutes.
**Total Prep Time:** 30 minutes

**Ingredients:**
- 1 lb beef sirloin, thinly sliced
- 2 tablespoons soy sauce
- 1 tablespoon oyster sauce
- 1 tablespoon hoisin sauce
- 1 tablespoon cornstarch
- 2 tablespoons vegetable oil
- 3 cups mixed vegetables (broccoli, bell peppers, snap peas)
- 2 cloves garlic, minced

- 1 tablespoon ginger, grated
- Green onions for garnish
- Sesame seeds for garnish
- Cooked rice for serving

## Instructions:

1. In a bowl, marinate sliced beef in soy sauce, oyster sauce, hoisin sauce, and cornstarch. Let it sit for 15 minutes.
2. Heat vegetable oil in a wok or skillet over high heat.
3. Add marinated beef and stir-fry until browned and cooked through. Remove from the wok and set aside.
4. In the same wok, add a bit more oil if needed. Stir-fry mixed vegetables, garlic, and ginger until vegetables are tender-crisp.
5. Return the cooked beef to the wok and toss everything together.
6. Garnish with green onions and sesame seeds.
7. Serve hot over cooked rice.
8. Enjoy Beef and Vegetable Stir-Fry.

## Nutritional Information: (Per Serving)

- Calories: 400
- Protein: 25g
- Carbohydrates: 20g
- Fat: 25g
- Fiber: 5g

# Stuffed Acorn Squash with Quinoa and Cranberries

**Intro:** Embrace the flavors of fall with Stuffed Acorn Squash with Quinoa and Cranberries. Nutty quinoa and sweet cranberries are stuffed inside roasted acorn squash halves, creating a wholesome and festive dish.

**Total Prep Time:** 1 hour

## Ingredients:
- 2 acorn squash, halved and seeds removed
- 1 cup quinoa, cooked
- 1/2 cup dried cranberries
- 1/2 cup pecans, chopped
- 1/4 cup fresh parsley, chopped
- 2 tablespoons olive oil
- 1 tablespoon maple syrup
- Salt and pepper to taste

## Instructions:
1. Preheat the oven to 375°F (190°C).
2. Place acorn squash halves on a baking sheet.
3. Brush the cut sides with olive oil and maple syrup. Season with salt and pepper.
4. Roast for 40-45 minutes or until the squash is fork-tender.
5. In a bowl, mix cooked quinoa, dried cranberries, chopped pecans, fresh parsley, and a drizzle of olive oil.
6. Fill each roasted acorn squash half with the quinoa mixture.
7. Serve warm and enjoy Stuffed Acorn Squash with Quinoa and Cranberries.

**Nutritional Information:** (Per Serving, 1/2 squash)
- Calories: 300
- Protein: 7g
- Carbohydrates: 55g
- Fat: 8g

- Fiber: 9g

# Lemon Garlic Shrimp with Asparagus

**Intro:** Brighten up your dinner with the zesty flavors of Lemon Garlic Shrimp with Asparagus. Succulent shrimp is sautéed with crisp asparagus in a lemony garlic butter sauce, creating a quick and delicious meal.
**Total Prep Time:** 20 minutes

## Ingredients:
- 1 lb large shrimp, peeled and deveined
- 1 lb asparagus, trimmed and cut into bite-sized pieces
- 3 tablespoons butter
- 3 cloves garlic, minced
- Zest and juice of 1 lemon
- 1/4 cup fresh parsley, chopped
- Salt and pepper to taste
- Cooked quinoa or rice for serving

## Instructions:
1. In a large pan, melt butter over medium heat.
2. Add shrimp and cook until pink and opaque.
3. Add asparagus, minced garlic, lemon zest, and lemon juice. Sauté until asparagus is tender-crisp.
4. Season with salt and pepper, and toss in fresh parsley.
5. Serve over cooked quinoa or rice.
6. Enjoy Lemon Garlic Shrimp with Asparagus.

## Nutritional Information: (Per Serving)
- Calories: 300
- Protein: 25g

- Carbohydrates: 10g
- Fat: 18g
- Fiber: 4g

## Sweet Potato and Chickpea Curry

**Intro:** Delight in the warm and comforting flavors of Sweet Potato and Chickpea Curry. This vegan-friendly dish combines tender sweet potatoes, hearty chickpeas, and aromatic spices in a luscious coconut curry sauce.
**Total Prep Time:** 45 minutes

### Ingredients:
- 2 large sweet potatoes, peeled and diced
- 1 can (15 oz) chickpeas, drained and rinsed
- 1 onion, finely chopped
- 2 cloves garlic, minced
- 1 can (14 oz) diced tomatoes
- 1 can (14 oz) coconut milk
- 2 tablespoons curry powder
- 1 teaspoon ground cumin
- 1 teaspoon ground coriander
- 1/2 teaspoon turmeric
- Salt and pepper to taste
- Fresh cilantro for garnish
- Cooked basmati rice for serving

### Instructions:
1. In a large pot, sauté onion and garlic until softened.
2. Add diced sweet potatoes, chickpeas, diced tomatoes, coconut milk, curry powder, cumin, coriander, turmeric, salt, and pepper.
3. Bring to a simmer and cook for 25-30 minutes or until sweet potatoes are tender.

4. Adjust seasoning as needed.
5. Serve over cooked basmati rice.
6. Garnish with fresh cilantro.
7. Enjoy Sweet Potato and Chickpea Curry.

**Nutritional Information:** (Per Serving)
- Calories: 400
- Protein: 10g
- Carbohydrates: 50g
- Fat: 20g
- Fiber: 12g

# Pesto Zucchini Noodles with Grilled Chicken

**Intro:** Indulge in a light and flavorful dish with Pesto Zucchini Noodles with Grilled Chicken. Zucchini noodles are tossed in a vibrant pesto sauce and topped with grilled chicken, creating a low-carb and delicious meal.
**Total Prep Time:** 30 minutes

**Ingredients:**
- 4 medium zucchinis, spiralized into noodles
- 1 lb chicken breasts, grilled and sliced
- 1 cup cherry tomatoes, halved
- 1/2 cup pine nuts, toasted
- 1/2 cup fresh basil leaves
- 2 cloves garlic, minced
- 1/2 cup Parmesan cheese, grated
- 1/2 cup extra-virgin olive oil
- Salt and pepper to taste
- Red pepper flakes for garnish
- Lemon wedges for serving

**Instructions:**
1. In a blender, combine basil, garlic, Parmesan cheese, and pine nuts. Blend until well combined.
2. With the blender running, slowly pour in the olive oil until a smooth pesto sauce forms. Season with salt and pepper.
3. In a large bowl, toss zucchini noodles with cherry tomatoes and half of the pesto sauce.
4. Top with grilled chicken slices.
5. Drizzle the remaining pesto sauce over the chicken.
6. Garnish with red pepper flakes and serve with lemon wedges.
7. Enjoy Pesto Zucchini Noodles with Grilled Chicken.

**Nutritional Information:** (Per Serving)
- Calories: 450
- Protein: 30g
- Carbohydrates: 10g
- Fat: 35g
- Fiber: 4g

## Baked Cod with Tomato and Olive Relish

**Intro:** Elevate your seafood dinner with Baked Cod with Tomato and Olive Relish. Tender cod fillets are baked to perfection and topped with a flavorful relish made from tomatoes, olives, and aromatic herbs.

**Total Prep Time:** 25 minutes

**Ingredients:**
- 4 cod fillets
- 1 cup cherry tomatoes, halved
- 1/2 cup Kalamata olives, pitted and sliced
- 3 tablespoons fresh parsley, chopped

- 2 tablespoons olive oil
- 1 tablespoon capers
- 2 cloves garlic, minced
- Salt and pepper to taste
- Lemon wedges for serving

**Instructions:**
1. Preheat the oven to 400°F (200°C).
2. Place cod fillets in a baking dish.
3. In a bowl, combine cherry tomatoes, Kalamata olives, fresh parsley, olive oil, capers, minced garlic, salt, and pepper.
4. Spoon the tomato and olive relish over the cod fillets.
5. Bake for 15-20 minutes or until the cod is opaque and flakes easily.
6. Garnish with additional fresh parsley.
7. Serve hot with lemon wedges.
8. Enjoy Baked Cod with Tomato and Olive Relish.

**Nutritional Information:** (Per Serving)
- Calories: 250
- Protein: 30g
- Carbohydrates: 5g
- Fat: 12g
- Fiber: 2g

# Quinoa and Spinach Stuffed Mushrooms

**Intro:** Enjoy a delightful appetizer or side dish with Quinoa and Spinach Stuffed Mushrooms. These bite-sized mushrooms are filled with a savory mixture of quinoa, spinach, and Parmesan cheese, making them a crowd-pleasing treat.

**Total Prep Time:** 40 minutes

**Ingredients:**
- 16 large white mushrooms, cleaned and stems removed
- 1 cup quinoa, cooked
- 2 cups fresh spinach, chopped
- 1/2 cup Parmesan cheese, grated
- 2 cloves garlic, minced
- 1 tablespoon olive oil
- Salt and pepper to taste
- Fresh parsley for garnish

**Instructions:**
1. Preheat the oven to 375°F (190°C).
2. In a pan, sauté garlic in olive oil until fragrant.
3. Add chopped spinach and cook until wilted.
4. In a bowl, combine cooked quinoa, sautéed spinach, Parmesan cheese, salt, and pepper.
5. Stuff each mushroom cap with the quinoa mixture.
6. Place stuffed mushrooms on a baking sheet.
7. Bake for 20-25 minutes or until mushrooms are tender.
8. Garnish with fresh parsley.
9. Serve warm and enjoy Quinoa and Spinach Stuffed Mushrooms.

**Nutritional Information:** (Per Serving, 4 mushrooms)
- Calories: 150
- Protein: 8g
- Carbohydrates: 20g
- Fat: 5g
- Fiber: 3g

# Butternut Squash and Sage Risotto

**Intro:** Delight your senses with the creamy and flavorful Butternut Squash and Sage Risotto. Arborio rice is cooked to perfection in a savory broth, then mixed with roasted butternut squash and fragrant sage.
**Total Prep Time:** 45 minutes

## Ingredients:
- 2 cups Arborio rice
- 1 butternut squash, peeled and diced
- 1 onion, finely chopped
- 3 cloves garlic, minced
- 4 cups vegetable broth, heated
- 1 cup dry white wine
- 1/2 cup Parmesan cheese, grated
- 3 tablespoons fresh sage, chopped
- 2 tablespoons butter
- Salt and pepper to taste

## Instructions:
1. Preheat the oven to 400°F (200°C).
2. Toss diced butternut squash with olive oil, salt, and pepper. Roast until tender.
3. In a large pot, sauté onion and garlic until softened.
4. Add Arborio rice and cook until lightly toasted.
5. Pour in the white wine and cook until mostly absorbed.
6. Begin adding the heated vegetable broth, one ladle at a time, stirring until absorbed before adding more.
7. Continue this process until the rice is creamy and cooked to al dente.

8. Fold in the roasted butternut squash, Parmesan cheese, fresh sage, and butter.
9. Season with salt and pepper.
10. Serve hot and enjoy Butternut Squash and Sage Risotto.

**Nutritional Information:** (Per Serving)
- Calories: 400
- Protein: 8g
- Carbohydrates: 70g
- Fat: 10g
- Fiber: 6g

## Greek Chicken Souvlaki Skewers

**Intro:** Transport your taste buds to the Mediterranean with Greek Chicken Souvlaki Skewers. Tender marinated chicken is threaded onto skewers and grilled to perfection, then served with a refreshing tzatziki sauce.
**Total Prep Time:** 30 minutes (plus marination time)

**Ingredients:**
- 1.5 lbs chicken breast, cut into cubes
- 1/4 cup olive oil
- 3 tablespoons lemon juice
- 3 cloves garlic, minced
- 1 teaspoon dried oregano
- 1 teaspoon dried thyme
- Salt and pepper to taste
- Cherry tomatoes for skewering
- Red onion, sliced, for skewering
- Tzatziki sauce for serving

**Instructions:**
1. In a bowl, whisk together olive oil, lemon juice, minced garlic, oregano, thyme, salt, and pepper.
2. Add chicken cubes to the marinade, coating them evenly. Marinate for at least 2 hours or overnight.
3. Preheat the grill.
4. Thread marinated chicken, cherry tomatoes, and red onion slices onto skewers.
5. Grill skewers for 12-15 minutes or until chicken is cooked through.
6. Serve with tzatziki sauce.
7. Enjoy Greek Chicken Souvlaki Skewers.

**Nutritional Information:** (Per Serving)
- Calories: 300
- Protein: 25g
- Carbohydrates: 10g
- Fat: 18g
- Fiber: 2g

# Lentil and Vegetable Curry

**Intro:** Embrace a plant-based delight with Lentil and Vegetable Curry. Hearty lentils and a medley of vegetables are simmered in a rich and aromatic curry sauce, creating a nourishing and satisfying dish.
**Total Prep Time:** 45 minutes

**Ingredients:**
- 1 cup dry lentils, rinsed
- 1 onion, finely chopped
- 2 cloves garlic, minced
- 1 bell pepper, diced
- 1 zucchini, diced

- 1 carrot, diced
- 1 can (14 oz) diced tomatoes
- 1 can (14 oz) coconut milk
- 2 tablespoons curry powder
- 1 teaspoon ground cumin
- 1 teaspoon ground coriander
- 1/2 teaspoon turmeric
- 1/2 teaspoon red pepper flakes (optional)
- Salt and pepper to taste
- Fresh cilantro for garnish
- Cooked rice or naan for serving

### Instructions:

1. In a large pot, sauté onion and garlic until softened.
2. Add diced bell pepper, zucchini, and carrot. Cook until vegetables are tender.
3. Stir in dry lentils, diced tomatoes, coconut milk, curry powder, cumin, coriander, turmeric, red pepper flakes (if using), salt, and pepper.
4. Bring to a simmer, cover, and cook for 25-30 minutes or until lentils are tender.
5. Adjust seasoning as needed.
6. Serve over cooked rice or with naan.
7. Garnish with fresh cilantro.
8. Enjoy Lentil and Vegetable Curry.

### Nutritional Information: (Per Serving)

- Calories: 350
- Protein: 18g
- Carbohydrates: 45g
- Fat: 12g
- Fiber: 15g

Printed in Great Britain
by Amazon